# 31 Days of Healing

## DEVOTIONS TO HELP YOU RECEIVE HEALING AND RECOVER QUICKLY

*by*
**Mark Brazee**

**Harrison House**
Tulsa, Oklahoma

12 11 10 09     15 14 13 12

*31 Days of Healing—*
*Devotions To Help You Receive Healing*
*and Recover Quickly*
ISBN 13: 978-1-57794-614-4
ISBN 10: 1-57794-614-6
Copyright © 2003 by Mark Brazee
Mark Brazee Ministries
P.O. Box 1870
Broken Arrow, Oklahoma 74013-1870

Published by Harrison House, Inc.
P.O. Box 35035
Tulsa, Oklahoma 74153

# INTRODUCTION

Suppose you went to the doctor to receive relief from pain or sickness and he told you, "I have a new wonder drug I'm going to prescribe for you. There are no side effects, and it's guaranteed to heal you of your condition. Not only that, but it will actually bring health to every part of your body, no matter what the problem or ailment! However, you have to faithfully take it exactly according to instructions."

After hearing that, I bet you'd listen very carefully as the doctor explained how to use this wonderful medicine. You'd want to take your prescription just as instructed so you could receive its full benefits!

You may say, "Well, that's a nice thought, but it's all hypothetical. There is no such wonder drug that can do all that."

I have some good news for you—that imaginary prescription isn't imaginary! The medicine that the Great Physician has provided for you does all that and more!

You see, God says that when you attend to His Word, it's actually life to you and health, or medicine, to your flesh. (Prov. 4:20-22.) When you take God's medicine according to His instructions, it goes to work in your body to drive out pain, sickness, and disease. And it doesn't stop until it's made you whole from the top of your head to the soles of your feet!

But in order to walk in divine health, you have to take your medicine every day according to the Great Physician's prescription. That's where this daily devotional comes in.

*31 Days of Healing* provides a daily dose of God's medicine for you to take as you're on your way to health and wholeness. Make sure you take your divine prescription as instructed. In other words, don't just read your daily dose and then forget about it as you go on your way. Read it over and over. Meditate on its truth until it's planted down in your spirit. Throughout the day, release your faith by saying the confession at the end of each devotion, out loud.

As you do so, faithfully acting on the Word you are learning, your health will improve. In fact, I believe it won't be the same at this time next month, but you'll see the effects of God's medicine at work in your body—making you healed, strong, and whole!

## *Take God's Medicine*

*My son, attend to my words; incline thine ear unto my sayings. Let them not depart from thine eyes; keep them in the midst of thine heart. For they are life unto those that find them, and health to all their flesh.* Proverbs 4:20-22

In the original Hebrew, this Scripture literally says that God's Word is medicine to our flesh. (A marginal note in my *King James Version* Bible substitutes the word *medicine* for the word *health*.) Now, think about this: What if someone invented a medication that could cure anything wrong with the human body? He'd be rich overnight! People would take that medicine diligently to make sure it worked. Well, if we'd just give God's promises on healing the same credibility we give the medicines developed by medical science, we would have 100 times the results!

(Now, I'm not against medical doctors. In fact, I have several doctors in my close family. Thank God for doctors! They keep people alive until those people discover there is a better way.)

God's words may be medicine to all our flesh, but just like other medicine, we have to take it. If we just put it on the shelf and look at it, it won't do us any good.

How do we take God's medicine? We hear it and hear it and hear it. Romans 10:17 says, "So then faith cometh by hearing, and hearing by the word of God." When we take the time to continually hear God's Word, our faith hooks up and releases God's power—and we rise up healed!

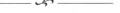

*Confession:*
*God's Word has the power to effect healing in my body.*
*I hear the Word and faith rises in me,*
*releasing God's power and producing what I need.*

## Don't Leave the Door Open!

*As the bird by wandering, as the swallow by flying, so the curse causeless shall not come.* Proverbs 26:2

If you were to leave the front door of your home wide open, any kind of animal—even a skunk—could walk right in. Spiritually speaking, Christians sometimes leave a "door" open to their lives for the enemy's "skunk" to enter.

Perhaps you're having trouble with obstacles the devil keeps throwing your way and you've done everything you know to do. Well, check to see if you've left a door open. By that I mean, for instance, are you walking in love? Are you harboring unforgiveness in your heart toward anyone?

You see, unforgiveness stops faith from working, because faith works by love, and love always forgives. (Gal. 5:6.) We may be trying to believe God for healing. But if we harbor unfor-giveness in our hearts, our faith will not work.

Sometimes people think they just can't forgive. They claim that the devil just won't let them. No, it isn't the devil who won't let people forgive; it's their own flesh—and the flesh can always be put under.

Forgiveness is not a feeling; it's a decision. We may have to reinforce that commitment to forgive again and again, but it's well worth the effort. When we keep all our doors shut, no skunks can get in to steal our blessings!

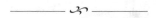

### Confession:

*I refuse to walk in unforgiveness and open the door to the devil. I won't allow the enemy's curse to come back on me. I choose to forgive, no matter what anyone does. I walk in love!*

## God Wants To Heal All

*And ye shall know the truth, and the truth shall make you free.*

*John 8:32*

People who say, "God doesn't heal anymore," evidently never read the Bible. Hebrews 13:8 says Jesus is the same now as He has ever been. If He healed while He walked on this earth, He still heals today.

Most people believe it is God's will to heal some. But the big question remains, "Is it God's will to heal all?" Some say, "Well, that can't be true because I knew Brother so-and-so, and he wasn't healed."

If we go by the experiences of people we know, we may conclude it isn't God's will to heal everyone. But we must gather together all the experience, tradition, doctrine, theory, and denominationalism we've ever heard and just push it aside. We must look at nothing but God's Word and find out what He has to say.

Let me illustrate. If you wanted to know my will about something, for example, I hope you wouldn't go ask some guy out on the street corner who doesn't know me. There's no telling what that person would say!

But most of us have done that with God. When we've wanted to know God's will, we've sometimes gone to people who don't even know Him and asked what they thought. They may have given us all kinds of wild opinions, not having the faintest idea what the Bible says.

So if we want to find God's will on a subject, we have to go to Jesus. He is the express image of God. Jesus said, "He that hath seen me hath seen the Father" (John 14:9). He also said, "And ye shall know the truth, and the truth shall make you free" (John 8:32). He didn't say theories or doctrines will make you free; He said knowing the truth—His Word—will make you free.

Thank God, the Bible is truth! And in the Bible, we find it is God's will to heal all.

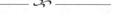

### Confession:

*I know the truth that God wants to heal me, and the truth sets me free from any sickness or disease. I've found it in the Word; I know it's God's will. So I believe I receive my healing now!*

## *Ask What You Will*

*If ye abide in me, and my words abide in you, ye shall ask*
*who ye will, and it shall be done unto you.* John 15:7

From this Scripture we understand that it is God's will to heal everyone, because it is God's will to answer prayers. God promises to answer any prayer that lines up with His Word.

We know that healing lines up with God's Word because Psalm 107:20 tells us God sent His Word to heal us. We know healing lines up with His Word because Matthew 9:35 tells us Jesus went through all the cities and villages, teaching, preaching, and healing every sickness and disease among the people. We know healing lines up with His Word because Hebrews 13:8 says Jesus is the same yesterday, today, and forever.

Jesus said, "If you abide in Me, and My words abide in you, you shall ask whatever you will, and it shall be done."

"Well, Lord, what if I will to be healed?" God's will is to heal you. And if healing is what you will, too, then you can be sure it shall be done unto you!

———— ✣ ————

*Confession:*

*I abide in the Lord Jesus Christ,*
*and His words abide in me.*
*So I ask my Father in prayer,*
*believing I receive my healing today.*
*By faith, it is done—I am healed!*

## First Hearing, Then Believing

*For whosoever shall call upon the name of the Lord shall be saved. How then shall they call on him in whom they have not believed? and how shall they believe in him of whom they have not heard? and how shall they hear without a preacher?*

*Romans 10:13,14*

Hearing the Word produces belief. You can't call on God unless you believe, and you can't believe unless you hear. That's why hearing and healing go hand in hand. Once you hear, you can believe; and once you believe, you can be healed.

Romans 10:17 says, "So then faith cometh by hearing, and hearing by the word of God." Hearing God's Word causes faith to rise up on the inside. When you release that faith, you get results. That's why Mark 9:23 says, "All things are possible to him that believeth."

God made it easy for you. He said simply to hear and be healed. So if you're having trouble believing God for your healing, don't try to work it up. Go back to the Word and "hear" what He said. Then just keep on hearing until faith rises up on the inside. Healing will be the result!

———— ✌ ————

### Confession:

*Because I hear the Word of God,
faith produces healing in my physical body.
Whosoever shall call upon the
name of the Lord shall be healed.
I hear, I call, I believe—and I am healed!*

## How To Receive From God

*Therefore I say unto you, What things soever ye desire, when ye pray, believe that ye receive them, and ye shall have them.*

Mark 11:24

How do we receive all that Jesus bought and paid for through His death, burial, and resurrection? Well, we know that faith operates on God's known will. So first we must look into the Word, where we find it's God's perfect will for every person to be born again and healed. Next, we make a point of contact, which occurs when we believe we receive—not necessarily when we see our petition come to pass.

Imagine a reservoir of water held back by a dam and a dry valley below. The two represent a "greater" and a "lesser"—a reservoir full of water and a valley that's dry. If you were to open the spillgate so that contact is made between the two, the greater would flood into the lesser.

In the same way, our point of contact can be likened to "opening the spillgate." The moment we release our faith—the point of contact—the greater anointing and power that is in Jesus Christ begins to flow into the "lesser," our bodies, whether we feel it or not. God's healing power begins to effect a healing in our physical bodies the moment we believe we receive.

In John 11:40, Jesus said to Martha, "I told you if you'd believe, you'd see the glory of God." Notice He didn't say, "I told you that when you see God's glory, then you'll believe."

Anyone can believe when he sees or feels something. But as Christians, we're supposed to believe we receive our answer before we see or feel it, because we believe the Word.

What else are we supposed to do? We are to say what we believe: "Thank God, I believe I'm healed by the stripes of Jesus." Do we necessarily feel any different? Not always, but that's all right. Our feelings won't change God's Word, but

God's Word will definitely change our feelings when we hook up with Him!

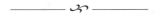

*Confession:*

*Today I make my point of contact with God.*
*By faith I open the spillgate of His goodness,*
*and His healing power flows into me*
*as I believe I receive!*

## *Remember All God Has Done for You*

*...and the soul of the people was much discouraged because of the way.*                    Numbers 21:4

As the children of Israel made their way toward the Promised Land, they became discouraged because they were looking at the way—the natural hardships of their journey.

But just think what they could have focused on instead. God had brought them out of Egypt with signs, wonders, and miracles. When they could go no farther because of the Red Sea, God had worked a miracle, parting the waters so they could cross on dry ground. When the Egyptian army had tried to pursue them, the two walls of water had closed up again and destroyed the Israelites' enemies.

When the Israelites had come to the waters of Marah, where the water was bitter, God had miraculously purified the waters so the people could have water to drink.

God led them with a pillar of cloud by day and a pillar of fire by night. He gave them fresh manna from heaven every night; all they had to do was pick it up. He even gave them water out of a rock. And for the entire forty years that the Israelites wandered through the desert, their shoes and clothes didn't wear out.

But, despite all of these things, the Israelites became discouraged because they looked at the way. We've done the same things at times. "Oh, Lord, things are so hard. The way is so tough. I feel so bad."

We need to look back in our lives and recognize how God has helped us—how He's brought us out of trials and delivered us from bondage. Realizing how much God has already done—and how much more He wants to do—for us, is an instant cure for discouragement!

———— ஃ ————

*Confession:*

*Through the blood of Jesus, my Father has delivered me, protected me, provided for me, and healed me. Therefore, no matter what I face, I focus my spiritual eyes on my faithful God.*

## *He Already Paid the Price*

*Giving thanks unto the Father, which hath made us meet to
be partakers of the inheritance of the saints in light.*

*Colossians 1:12*

Jesus went to the cross and shed His blood for
us. Through His death, burial, and resurrection, He forgave our sins, redeemed us, delivered
us from the power of darkness, and enabled us
to become partakers of God's inheritance.

Yet most Christians have had a very low
opinion of what redemption really is. They will
say, "Well, Jesus redeemed me from sin."

That's true, but there's so much more to it.
Thank God, we've been redeemed from every
curse in the Old Testament—and that includes
sickness!

Now, Jesus didn't redeem us from all the Old
Testament blessings. For instance, healing was a

blessing back then, so it's still a blessing today. Jesus didn't do away with any blessings; He just added to them.

Look at Isaiah 53:5: "But he was wounded for our transgressions, he was bruised for our iniquities: the chastisement of our peace was upon him; and with his stripes we are healed." Jesus not only redeemed us from our sins, but He also redeemed us from torment and oppression so we could have peace. He redeemed us from sickness so we could have health.

God's report says we were forgiven, delivered, and healed. Now we can just reach out in faith to receive any of these covenant blessings. They all belong to us because Jesus already paid the price.

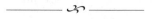

*Confession:*

*I am free from sin and all its effects—from worry, anxiety, and fear, from sickness, disease, and pain. God's inheritance affects all areas of my life—spirit, soul, and body.*

## *Let Patience Have Her Perfect Work*

*My brethren, count it all joy when ye fall into divers tempta-*
*tions; knowing this, that the trying of your faith worketh*
*patience. But let patience have her perfect work, that ye may*
*be perfect and entire, wanting nothing.*        James 1:2-4

Notice in verse 4 that James didn't say, "Let those tests and trials have their perfect work." He said, "Let patience have her perfect work...."

You see, tests and trials don't perfect you. It is what you do with them that counts. You are not perfected because a bunch of problems come along. You are perfected because you stick with the Word of God in the midst of those problems and patiently endure. That's when patience has its perfect work.

Patience is consistent endurance. When you walk in patience, you remain consistent all the way through situations, no matter what comes along. You aren't up and down like a yo-yo. You base everything on God's Word. You don't get up in the morning and ask yourself how you are. You get up in the morning, open your Bible, and tell yourself how you are according to the Word!

I've seen people grow in their spiritual walks as a result of using their faith against tests and trials. I've seen other people go under when they faced the same tests and trials. It's what people do with their problems that makes the difference.

Faith thrives in the midst of a trial. That doesn't mean we enjoy the trial. But when it comes our way, we don't shrink away from it either! We stand on God's Word and say, "Thank God, I know and trust the One whom I have believed!" Even when the going gets tough, we just dig our heels in and say, "I don't care what it looks like, seems like, sounds like, or feels like. I believe what the Word of God says!"

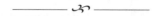

*Confession:*

*My faith thrives in the midst of a trial.*
*When symptoms come, I tell my body,*
*"You're healed because Jesus bore your sickness!"*
*I'm not the sick trying to get healed. I am the healed,*
*and in Jesus' name the symptoms have to leave!*

## Come Out of the Trial Stronger!

*Fight the good fight of faith, lay hold on eternal life, whereunto thou art also called, and hast professed a good profession before many witnesses.* 1 Timothy 6:12

Someone said, "I thought when a person operated in faith, he wouldn't have any problems." No, that's what faith is for—to help you overcome the enemy when he attacks you with problems.

A man came to one minister and said, "I want you to pray I'll never have any more trouble with the devil."

The minister said, "Do you want me to pray you will die?"

You can count on it—the enemy will come with tests and trials. He is trying to steal, kill, and destroy everything good in your life.

(John 10:10.) As long as we live down here, we will have trouble with the devil.

What does the devil do? He tries to stir up negative circumstances, symptoms, thoughts, imaginations, and trials. He does anything he can to discourage us and make us quit. I'm not preaching doom and gloom; I'm just saying we may as well face the fact that life on this earth won't be "a bed of roses."

Even though we are Christians, problems will come to us in life. But we aren't supposed to hide, bury our heads in the sand, or run in fear and cry, "Oh, God, what am I going to do now?"

We just need to stay scriptural. Then every time symptoms, temptations, tests, or trials come along, we'll get a silly grin on our faces and say, "Glory to God! Here's one more chance for me to flex my faith muscles. I'll come out of this stronger. The next time the devil comes, he'd better have some bigger guns because whatever he throws against me, I'm throwing back in his face with the Word of God! And in the name of Jesus, I'll grow as a result of it!"

—————— ꝛ ——————

*Confession:*

*I overcome every test, every trial, and every symptom*
*with God's Word and the name of Jesus.*
*I will not be discouraged,*
*I will not fear, and I will not quit.*
*I come out of every test stronger*
*because I am growing in faith!*

## Be a Doer of the Word

*This book of the law shall not depart out of thy mouth; but thou shalt meditate therein day and night, that thou mayest observe to do according to all that is written therein: for then thou shalt make thy way prosperous, and then thou shalt have good success.*  Joshua 1:8

I f you want to walk in divine health, as God desires, you have to be a doer of the Word. For one thing, that means meditating on God's healing promises. As you do, you'll find His Word getting so big on the inside that you start acting like a healthy person!

God told Joshua the results he could expect for being diligent in His Word: "For then thou shalt make thy way prosperous, and then thou shalt have good success." Did you notice that it doesn't say, "For then God will make your way prosperous"? No, it says, "For you will make your way prosperous." I've also heard it put this way—"Then you will deal wisely in all the affairs of life."

God has made health and success available in every area of your life. Now He says, "I give you the wisdom and ability to deal wisely in all the affairs of life. But it's your choice whether or not you become a doer of My Word and actually receive what I've given you."

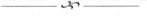

*Confession:*
*I have planted God's Word in my heart, and that Word is life to me and health to all my flesh. Because I meditate on God's Word, I deal wisely in all the affairs of life.*

## *It Pays To Persevere*

*Then came she and worshipped him, saying, Lord, help me.*
*But he answered and said, It is not meet to take the chil-*
*dren's bread, and to cast it to dogs. And she said, Truth,*
*Lord: yet the dogs eat of the crumbs which fall from their*
*masters' table. Then Jesus answered and said unto her, O*
*woman, great is thy faith: be it unto thee even as thou wilt.*
*And her daughter was made whole from that very hour.*
*Matthew 15:25-28*

Under similar circumstances most of us
would have given up, but not this woman.
First Jesus ignored her; then He said to His disciples, "I'm not even sent to help her." Still, "came
she and worshipped him, saying, Lord, help me."
This Gentile mother wouldn't leave Jesus alone!

Then Jesus told her it wasn't right to take the
children's bread and give it to dogs. Jesus called
her a dog! Most of us would have gone home
angry. But look what she told Jesus: "Truth, Lord:

yet the dogs eat of the crumbs which fall from their masters' table."

You may have thought she responded that way because of her humble attitude. "O Lord, just give me one of the crumbs from Your table!" But she was really saying, "Lord, I don't need the whole loaf. Give that to the children, although most of them won't take it. Just give me a crumb. I know what Your bread will do."

She was not talking about how much humility she had; she was talking about how powerful Jesus' bread is! She was saying, "Call me anything you want to, but heal my daughter."

Then Jesus told her, "With faith like that, you can have anything you want!" Jesus had taken this woman to the limits, and she'd passed the test. He knew her faith would turn His power loose.

Great faith always takes God at His Word, and that's what this Gentile woman did. It paid to hang on and refuse to give up, because she received the answer she'd come for: Her daughter was made whole!

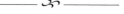

*Confession:*

*I hold fast to God's Word with tenacity until my healing is manifested. I refuse to give up, because I know that God's Word works!*

## *Take a Stand!*

*And a certain woman, which had an issue of blood twelve years, ...came in the press behind, and touched his garment.*

Mark 5:25,27

The more you consider this woman with the issue of blood, the more you understand that she had to be stubborn. Under the Jewish law, she was considered unclean. When a woman with an issue of blood came out in public, she risked being stoned.

As if that weren't bad enough, notice whom Jesus was walking with at the time: "And, behold, there cometh one of the rulers of the synagogue, Jairus by name" (v. 22).

Jesus was on His way to Jairus's house to heal his daughter when He perceived that power had flowed out of Him and stopped to find out who had touched Him. As a ruler of the synagogue, Jairus had authority to have this woman stoned.

This woman had to be tenacious, stubborn, resistant to flow. She had to overcome her fear and go against religious leaders.

You know, some ministers say, "Well, you just can't be healed. God doesn't do that anymore." When that happens, people have to override what those ministers are saying about healing in order to receive their healing.

This woman had to overcome unbelief, fear, and weakness. She had to decide that no matter what came against her, she was going to receive her healing.

We have to get to that same point and make the same decision: "I don't care what anyone says. I don't care what it looks like, seems like, or feels like. I'm taking a stand on God's Word, and that's all there is to it!"

———— ❧ ————

## Confession:

*I will not be moved by circumstances or
by what others say about my situation.
I am moved only by what God's Word says.
No sickness is too hard for my Father to heal.
I receive my healing today!*

## *Act in Faith as God Leads You*

*When he [Jesus] had thus spoken, he spat on the ground, and made clay of the spittle, and he anointed the eyes of the blind man with the clay, and said unto him, Go, wash in the pool of Siloam, (which is by interpretation, Sent.) He went his way therefore, and washed, and came seeing.*

*John 9:6,7*

You may wonder, *What should I do to act on my faith?*

Don't do something because it worked for someone else. Let God show you how to act in faith.

Jesus spit in the dirt, made clay of the spittle, put it on a blind man's eyes, and said, "Go wash in the pool of Siloam." (John 9:6,7.) But He didn't tell anyone else to go dip in that pool. Jesus gave people a whole variety of instructions for acting on their faith.

I had a friend who was waiting for God to heal him from severe sugar diabetes. He heard of someone who had thrown away his insulin, so he thought, *That's my step of faith! If I throw away this insulin, God will have to do something.* But the man almost died! He tried to make something happen instead of acting because he believed God had already healed him.

Another time, I traveled for a summer with a group that included two people who had sugar diabetes. I watched these people throughout the summer. They had to check the amount of insulin they needed every day. Every time they checked, they said, "Thank You, Father. I believe I'm healed by Jesus' stripes. Glory to God!" Then they'd take whatever insulin they needed.

The insulin wasn't healing these two people; it was just keeping them alive. A week or so later, they'd need a little bit less insulin. They'd take whatever insulin they needed, but they'd always say, "Thank God, I believe I'm healed."

Over a period of about three months, I watched both of these people get healed of diabetes. By the end of the summer, neither one of them needed any insulin!

So let God teach you what you need to do to act on your faith. Then obey Him, and be healed!

———— ✺ ————

*Confession:*

*God shows me how to act in faith,*
*and I follow His instructions and*
*praise Him because His Word is true!*

# *Keep the Law of Love*

*And hope maketh not ashamed; because the love of God is shed abroad in our hearts by the Holy Ghost which is given unto us.*                                    Romans 5:5

One way for us to stay healthy is to walk in love.

Under the old covenant, God told His people that if they served Him, He would take sickness away from the midst of them. (Ex. 23:25.) Then He gave His people a list of commandments and ordinances to obey, knowing that the Israelites had no power to fulfill them.

In essence, He was saying to them, "Here are all these rules and regulations to follow in order to live holy before Me. However, there's no way you can keep them. So when you break My laws, the blood of an animal sacrifice will cover your sins and iniquities. It will push your sins ahead for a year so you can receive My blessings."

God gave His laws and commandments to His people to prove to them that they needed a Savior. Galatians 3:24 says the law served as a schoolmaster to bring God's people to Jesus. God's people couldn't be perfected through the Law. They needed a Redeemer.

What about us? Are we in better shape today? Are we able to obey Jesus' commandment to "Love one another" (John 13:34) any better than the Old Testament saints were able to keep the Law?

Under the old covenant, God's people possessed the Law but had no power to keep it. Under the new covenant, when we're born again, the Holy Ghost indwells us and imparts the love of God into our spirits. We then have the power to keep the law of love. And as long as we walk in love, we have the power to fulfill the other commandments as well.

So, actually, our job on this earth is to walk in love. As long as we walk in love, we're keeping

God's commandments. And as long as we keep His commandments, our God, Jehovah Rapha, will take sickness from the midst of us!

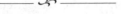

### Confession:

*God's love is shed abroad in my heart.*
*God, my Healer, heals me and keeps me*
*in divine health as I follow the ways*
*of His Word and His Spirit.*

## *Don't Deny the Problem*

*And being not weak in faith, he [Abraham] considered not his own body now dead, when he was about an hundred years old, neither yet the deadness of Sarah's womb.*

*Romans 4:19*

Did you notice that Abraham never denied the problem? He just didn't consider it. He never said, "No, I'm not 100 years old. I'm more like 20 or 25."

God doesn't want us to deny that the problem exists. He doesn't advocate lying or "mind over matter." He's just saying, "You can look at the problem, but don't consider it. Switch over and consider the Word. Don't deny that the problem is there; just observe the Word. Keep your eyes on the answer."

I once overheard someone say to another person, "Oh, you look sick! You look like you have a cold."

The other person replied, "No, I don't. I'm not sick."

The first person said, "Well, your nose is running."

"No, it isn't."

"But you sound sick."

"No, I'm not sick," the second person insisted. But everyone around him could see he was sick. This person thought he was in faith, but he was just denying the problem.

God doesn't want us to do that. He just wants us to say, "It doesn't matter what I look like, feel like, or sound like. The only thing that matters is what God says. God tells me that by Jesus' stripes I was healed, and I've chosen to believe Him!"

So don't deny the problem or try to think it away. Just look at it and say, "Who cares? The answer is mine—I have God's Word on it!"

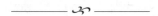

*Confession:*

*I don't deny the problems that arise in my life.
I just believe God's Word, which is greater than
any symptoms, circumstances, or problems.
I am fully persuaded that what God
has promised, He is able to do.*
*(Rom. 4:21.)*

## *In Remembrance*

*The Lord Jesus the same night in which he was betrayed took bread: And when he had given thanks, he brake it, and said, Take, eat: this is my body, which is broken for you: this do in remembrance of me. After the same manner also he took the cup, when he had supped, saying, this cup is the new testament in my blood: this do ye, as oft as ye drink it, in remembrance of me. For as often as ye eat this bread, and drink this cup, ye do shew the Lord's death till he come.*                    *1 Corinthians 11:23-26*

In Exodus 12, God told His people, who were living in bondage in Egypt, "Slay a spotless lamb and put its blood on the doorposts; then roast the lamb and eat it. But before you do, pack your bags, put your marching shoes on, and get ready to travel, because after you partake of the lamb, you're coming out of this bondage."

As the Israelites ate the body of that Passover lamb, they looked ahead to the redemptive work that would be accomplished when Jesus Christ went to the cross. Under the new covenant, we take Communion to look back and remember what Jesus did for us.

We once were trapped in the bondage of sickness, worry, fear, discouragement, and depression. But the perfect Lamb shed His blood to redeem us from every yoke of bondage. Therefore, God's message to us is similar to what He said to the Israelites in Egypt. He says to us, "When you partake of the symbols of the body of the Lord Jesus Christ, put your marching shoes on and get ready to come out of bondage!"

Communion services should be some of the biggest healing rallies around. When we partake of Communion, we remember what Jesus Christ did for us. For instance, we partake of the bread in remembrance of Jesus' body, broken for our physical healing. Therefore, we should say, "Thank You, Jesus, that by Your shed blood on the cross, my sins were washed away. By Your broken body, I've been healed. And by Your chastisement, I have peace of mind." (Isa. 53:5.)

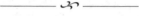

*Confession:*
*On the cross, Jesus freed my spirit, soul, and body from all bondage. Now I partake of Communion, believing I'm freed from sin and sickness because of His finished work.*

## Faith Turns God Loose!

*And, behold, there cometh one of the rulers of the syna-
gogue, Jairus by name; and when he saw him, he fell at his
feet, And besought him greatly, saying, My little daughter
lieth at the point of death: I pray thee, come and lay thy
hands on her, that she may be healed; and she shall live.
And Jesus went with him....*                    Mark 5:22-24

Jesus started walking with Jairus toward his
house. About that time, the woman with the
issue of blood came up behind Him in the
crowd and touched the hem of His garment.
Jesus turned and asked, "Who touched Me?" The
woman fell down before Jesus and told Him how
she had been healed. (Mark 5:25-33.)

All this was going on while Jairus's daughter
was at home at the point of death. When Jesus
finished with the woman, they all started again
toward Jairus's house. But just then someone
came running from Jairus's home and told him,

"It's too late. Don't trouble the Master; your daughter has died."

Jesus immediately turned to Jairus and made a profound statement: "Fear not; only believe." At that moment, He laid out a choice before Jairus, telling him, "You're either going to fear, or you're going to believe. If you keep operating in faith, your child will be healed. But if you step over into fear, you shut off My power."

You see, our words can open the door for the devil to attack us. Proverbs 6:2 says, "Thou art snared with the words of thy mouth, thou art taken with the words of thy mouth." Fear allows Satan to work in our lives. It often starts out with worry, which is an offspring of fear, and that turns the devil loose.

When Jairus first found Jesus, he had spoken words of faith: "Jesus, if You lay hands on her, she will be healed and live." Now Jesus was giving him a choice, and Jairus chose to believe. He didn't speak one word of doubt or fear, and his little girl was raised from the dead. His faith turned God loose to work in his daughter's life.

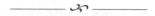

*Confession:*
*I refuse to allow fear to operate in my life.*
*I make the choice to walk in faith.*
*I speak words of life and truth that open*
*the door for God to make me healthy and whole!*

## The End Result

*Now a certain man was sick, named Lazarus, of Bethany,
the town of Mary and her sister Martha. Therefore his
sisters sent unto him, saying, Lord, behold, he whom thou
lovest is sick. When Jesus heard that, he said, This sickness
is not unto death, but for the glory of God, that the Son of
God might be glorified thereby.*          John 11:1,3,4

Don't misunderstand Jesus' comment about
Lazarus' sickness. He was not saying,
"Lazarus' sickness isn't unto death; neverthe-
less, he's suffering with this sickness to bring
God glory."

If we're not careful, we can get confused
because we don't study the Word enough to
rightly divide it. Jesus wasn't talking about the
problem; He was talking about the end result.
Jesus always talked about the end result. He was
saying here, "The end result of this sickness will
not be death but the glory of God."

Again in John 11:40, Jesus told Martha, "I told you if you'd believe, you'd see the glory of God." The sickness took Lazarus' life for a while, but his life was given back to him when Jesus raised him from the dead. Thus, Lazarus' sickness wasn't for God's glory; it was his resurrection from the dead that brought God glory. That was the end result.

—— ॐ ——

*Confession:*

*God is glorified when I am healed*
*and walking in health.*
*The end result of my life will be to God's glory.*
*I walk in health and run my race,*
*and I will finish my course with joy!*

## The Connection Between Saying and Believing

*We having the same spirit of faith, according as it is written, I believed, and therefore have I spoken; we also believe, and therefore speak.* 2 Corinthians 4:13

I heard a minister say, "Anytime you see a there-fore in the Bible, stop and see what it's there for." In this verse, Paul uses the word *therefore* to combine the two parts of faith: "I believed and therefore have I spoken; we also believe, and therefore speak."

If we're going to believe something, we also have to speak it. Believing alone doesn't make it come to pass. It has to be combined with saying what God's Word says.

Jesus said, "If you believe in your heart that what you say will come to pass, you'll have whatever you say." (Mark 11:23.) The truth is, we can spend a lot of time feeding on God's Word, but what we continually say is what we'll ultimately believe.

When I was growing up, I had a friend who was a chronic liar. He started out lying just to get himself out of trouble, but it eventually became a habit. He'd make up a whopper of a lie about some situation; then six months later, no one could convince him it hadn't happened that way. He'd said the lie so much that he actually believed it.

If that can be done with a lie, we should be able to do the same thing with the truth of God's Word. When we first start saying, "By Jesus' stripes I was healed," it can sound hollow. It's easy to think, I know the Bible says that by His stripes I was healed, but I feel sick from head to toe. But as we keep saying it and saying it, soon we'll believe it no matter what we feel like.

How do you come to that place of faith? By feeding on God's Word and speaking it with your mouth. Once you believe in your heart what God says, you can declare it with the added push of faith behind your words. Then get ready, for your answer will come to pass!

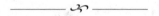

## Confession:

*God's Word is truth. As I continually speak
His Word and believe it with my heart,
His Word becomes truth in me. I believe God's truth,
I declare God's truth, and I receive His very best!*

## *Seek Healing, Not Sympathy*

*Let us hold fast the profession of our faith without*
*wavering; (for he is faithful that promised).*

*Hebrews 10:23*

Notice that this verse talks about holding fast to your profession of faith. You know, if you have to hold fast to something, it usually means it's trying to get away from you. You'll find in life that one of the most difficult things to hold fast to is the confession of your faith.

Folks will say to you, "You look terrible. How do you feel? I know what you believe, but how do you feel?" It's so tempting to switch over into the natural realm and just spew it all out, telling people how bad you really feel, how bad it looks, and how bad the doctor's report says it's going to get. Flesh just likes to get down and wallow in that mire of doubt and self-pity, looking for sympathy.

But I'd rather have healing than sympathy. Sympathy feels good for a few seconds, but healing feels good for a long time. I can hold fast to my symptoms and get sympathy. But I'd rather hold fast to my confession of faith and get results!

———— ❦ ————

*Confession:*
*Jesus was faithful to heal those*
*who came to Him in faith,*
*and He's still the same today.*
*I hold fast to my confession that I am healed*
*because faithful is He who has promised!*

## *What Do Your Words Carry?*

*The words of a wise man's mouth are gracious; but the lips of a fool will swallow up himself.*  Ecclesiastes 10:12

Our words create an atmosphere. Words are powerful "carriers"; they carry faith, or they carry unbelief. And whatever we fill our words with will directly affect our lives.

Sit down sometime and take a look at your life. You'll find things you do like. But if you look hard enough, you'll find some aspects of your life you don't like. Then ask yourself, "What have I been saying about those parts of my life that I don't like?"

If you don't like where you are in life, change your words. Quit saying what you're saying. Proverbs 18:21 says, "Death and life are in the power of the tongue...."

For instance, have you ever said, "I never get anything from God. I tried that faith stuff, but it didn't work for me"? If so, switch over to speaking words of faith: "I've been feeding on God's Word for years, and my faith is growing exceedingly. God's Word is seed planted in my heart, and it's working mightily in me!"

We are a direct result of what we've believed and said about ourselves in the past. So to make sure our future is different than our past or present, we often have to go back to the Bible and get our minds renewed and our thinking straightened out.

Once you get your thinking lined up with God's Word, it's amazing how easily your believing will line up right behind it. And after you get your believing straightened out, your mouth will straighten out! Out of the abundance of your heart, your mouth will begin to speak faith. (Matt. 12:34.)

You're in good shape when you have your thinking, believing, and speaking all lined up with God's Word. You're ready for your faith-filled words to carry you straight into a future of health and abundance!

———— ॐ ————

## Believe the Word, Not the Symptoms

*For we walk by faith, not by sight.*     2 Corinthians 5:7

I once heard about a lady who was a member of a particular church and had a big, visible, cancerous growth on her face. Apparently she made a point of contact, praying and believing she received her healing. But there was no change in her appearance.

Later at a testimony service, this woman stood and said, "I want to thank God for healing me." She sat down, and people started looking at her funny. The next Sunday, she stood and said, "I want to thank God for healing me." This went on for several weeks.

Some people got upset about it, and one person said to her, "Everyone can see you're not healed. You're causing confusion. You can't keep standing up telling people you're healed."

She went home that day and stood in front of the mirror. Then she prayed, "Now, Father, in Jesus' name, I know I'm healed by the stripes of Jesus. I know what the Bible says, and I know I believe it. I'd sure appreciate it, though, if You'd get rid of these ugly symptoms." All of a sudden, while the woman was still standing in front of the mirror, that big cancer just fell off and hit the floor! She looked in the mirror. The area where the growth had been a moment before was now covered in fresh baby skin!

When we make a point of contact with God, believing we receive our answer, we may not immediately look different. But we don't have to look different—we just have to believe what the Bible says and then say what we believe!

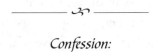

### Confession:

*Thank God, I'm healed! I know in my heart that when I prayed, my Father heard me and gave me the petition I asked for. I believe I have received my healing.*

## *Take Care of Your Temple*

*...that ye may be able to withstand in the evil day, and
having done all, to stand.*       Ephesians 6:13

Sometimes the reason we're experiencing
difficulty getting rid of sickness in our
bodies is that we've left a door open some-
place. Either we're doing something wrong, or
we're not doing something right. This isn't a
hard-and-fast rule, because the devil will still
try to attack when we're doing everything
right. But sometimes we will find we left a
door open.

For instance, I was a youth minister in
Colorado for about thirteen months. I lived in a
couple's home, and the wife was an amazing
cook. I gained about twenty-five pounds.

But then life got very busy. I had an opportunity to minister in two different schools,
and I was on a flat run all the time. For a

couple of months, I ate a lot of very unhealthy junk food. All of a sudden, my stomach started giving me trouble.

Now, I'm not a nervous, high-strung person. But when I tried to eat, I'd almost get sick to my stomach. My stomach just burned all the time. I had unknowingly opened the door for the devil to bring me stomach problems.

I prayed, "Lord, I'm sorry. My body is the temple of the Holy Ghost, and I've been misusing it. Lord, I repent." Then I believed I received my healing and got healed instantly.

So don't mistreat your body and leave a door open for the devil to bring in sickness and disease. Eat right and get adequate rest and exercise. Never forget—you are the custodian of the Holy Spirit's dwelling place!

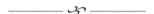

*Confession:*

*My body is the temple of the Holy Ghost.*
*I am the one responsible for taking care of it.*
*So I purpose to eat the proper diet, get plenty*
*of exercise and rest, and allow my body to*
*function according to God's design.*

## *Keep Your Eyes on the Answer*

*Then on the third day Abraham lifted up his eyes, and saw the place afar off. And Abraham said unto his young men, Abide ye here with the ass; and I and the lad will go yonder and worship, and come again to you.* Genesis 22:4,5

If you always have your eyes on the answer and consider only what God said, you'll overcome in the end, regardless of your situation. A good example of this principle is the story of Abraham.

Abraham's miracle child, Isaac, was born to him and Sarah because they "staggered not" at God's promise. But Isaac wasn't the fulfillment of the promise; he was just the means to the fulfillment of the promise. God didn't say, "I'll give you a son." He said, "I have made you the father of many nations. Your seed shall be numbered as the sands of the sea and the stars of the sky." (Gen. 17:4; 22:17.)

But in Genesis 22, God told Abraham to offer Isaac as a burnt offering to Him. Abraham would have been in trouble if he'd been walking around saying, "I know I'm the father of many nations because I have a son." If he had been thinking that way, he would have responded, "Lord, I can't do that. Isaac has to live, or I can't be the father of many nations."

But Abraham was absolutely convinced God's promise had to come to pass. He believed that if he sacrificed his son, God would have to raise him from the dead to fulfill that promise. (Heb. 11:17-19.) So Abraham told the servants, "I and the lad will go yonder and worship, and come again to you." He was saying, "Both of us will go up, and both of us will come back." And both of them did!

Don't take your eyes off the answer—off Jesus and the Word—for anything, whether good or bad. Even when your body is feeling better, don't dwell on that. Keep your eyes fixed on

God's promises. Say, "I know I'm healed, not because I feel good, but because the Bible says, 'By Jesus' stripes, I was healed.'"

Always keep your attention fixed on the eternal promises of God, not on the temporal circumstances of this world. Be fully persuaded that what God promised you will see come to pass!

———— ᔕ ————

*Confession:*
*Whether my body feels good or bad,*
*I keep my attention focused on God's healing promises.*
*Situations and circumstances must change,*
*but the Word will never change!*

## *Follow God's Instructions*

*And be not conformed to this world: but be ye transformed by the renewing of your mind, that ye may prove what is that good, and acceptable, and perfect, will of God.*

*Romans 12:2*

In order for the Word to work successfully, we must be sure we're following God's instructions. Many times people are deceived because they only attempt to stand on the Word and believe God for their healing. I remember some of my own early experiences. I attempted to stand on the Word. But when I first endeavored to believe for God to heal me of the flu, the sickness didn't go away for about seven days.

All that time, I knew if I were to let the sickness run its own course, it would also take about seven days. This frustrated me, until one day I realized I'd been doing something wrong. I'd been standing on the right Scriptures. I had them all located and memorized, but the Scriptures weren't planted on the inside of me. I had some head knowledge, but my heart hadn't grasped what the Word was really saying.

What's the solution to "head knowledge faith"? Read the Word, study the Word, meditate on the Word, and confess the Word—and keep on doing it! It takes time and work to believe what God says in the face of obstacles.

It's so important to make sure the Word goes from the mental realm to your heart! As a matter of fact, the difference between victory and defeat in the Christian life is the eighteen inches between your head and your heart. Do you just mentally agree with the Word, or is the Word planted in your heart? The answer to that question determines whether or not the Word will work for you.

As long as we live in this world, problems are going to come. That's all the more reason to do what God said: "Go to the Word." Grasp it, believe it, and then watch the Word go into action. God watches over His Word to perform it! (Jer. 1:12.)

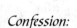

*Confession:*

*I renew my mind with the Word*
*and think God's thoughts.*
*His Word is planted and rooted*
*deep inside my heart.*
*No matter what obstacle I face, I believe*
*God's Word is true, and it changes my life!*

## Watch Your Attitude Before God

*And he [Jesus] spake this parable unto certain which*
*trusted in themselves that they were righteous, and despised*
*others: Two men went up into the temple to pray; the one a*
*Pharisee, and the other a publican. The Pharisee stood and*
*prayed thus with himself, God, I thank thee, that I am not*
*as other men are, extortioners, unjust, adulterers, or even as*
*this publican. I fast twice in the week, I give tithes of all*
*that I possess. And the publican, standing afar off, would*
*not lift up so much as his eyes unto heaven, but smote upon*
*his breast, saying, God be merciful to me a sinner.*

*Luke 18:9-13*

I believe Jesus is trying to show us the difference between the two men's attitudes here.
The Pharisee arrogantly boasted, "I do this and
that and everything else, God; Your blessings
belong to me now." The other man just humbly
prayed, "Lord, I don't deserve anything on my
own. Please just be merciful to me."

It's true we need to stand up in our righteousness. We are to come boldly before the throne of grace, believe and confess the Word and act in faith. Proverbs 28:1 says, "The righteous are bold as a lion."

But we shouldn't come with an arrogant attitude, saying, "God, I'm doing everything You said to do; You owe me."

We need to come and say, "Lord, I'm doing what You said in Your Word. Now I thank You for Your mercy."

God's mercy, compassion, and grace provided everything we have in Jesus Christ, and we must treat His blessings as a gift. Because of God's grace poured out upon us, we can say, "If we believe and say what His Word says, it will come to pass." We are to be thankfully receptive, not arrogant about it.

So be bold when you go before God, but always keep a watch on your attitude. Remember, it's only by God's grace that you stand!

———— ∾ ————

*Confession:*

*I go boldly before God's throne to receive my healing.*
*I don't deserve it on my own. But, praise God,*
*Jesus gave me His own right standing*
*with the Father so I could receive it.*

## Control Your Mouth–
## Control Your Life

*For we all often stumble and fall and offend in many things. And if anyone does not offend in speech [never says the wrong things], he is a fully developed character and a perfect man, able to control his whole body and to curb his entire nature.*                    James 3:2 (AMP)

The truth is, we've all made mistakes. But in the last part of this verse, James says, "If you can control your mouth, you can control your body and your entire nature." That's a strong statement!

In verse 3 (AMP), James gives us more information about the tongue: "If we set bits in the horses' mouths to make them obey us, we can turn their whole bodies about." Now, I'm not a horseman, but I know horses are too big to grab around the neck and pull around wherever you want. However, if you can put a bit in a horse's mouth, you can control the direction it goes.

James continues: "Likewise, look at the ships: though they are so great and are driven by rough winds, they are steered by a very small rudder wherever the impulse of the helmsman determines" (v. 4 AMP). Ships are big, and winds are strong. But when you control the rudder, you control where the ship goes.

Think about it this way: A horse wants to go a particular direction by its own inner will. A ship has no will, but outside forces, such as the wind and waves, try to drive it. So, putting a bit in a horse's mouth and directing a ship by its rudder are examples of controlling both inside desires and outside forces.

Apply this to your own life. The problem you face may come from within—a resistant will, the lusts of the flesh, and so forth. Or outside forces, such as symptoms of sickness, may be coming against you. Either way, the principle holds true:

As you control your mouth, you can control yourself—inside and out!

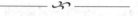

*Confession:*
*By the words of my mouth, I control the*
*direction of my life. I speak only what*
*God says about me and my circumstances,*
*so I'm headed straight toward victory!*

## A Treasure Hidden for Us

*And he taught them many things by parables, and said
unto them in his doctrine, Hearken; Behold, there went out
a sower to sow.*                                   Mark 4:2,3

I n this passage, Jesus began teaching a crowd
in parables. Later, when He was alone with
His disciples, they asked Him the meaning of the
parable of the sower. In essence they said, "We
don't understand what You're talking about."

Jesus said to them, "Unto you it is given to
know the mystery of the kingdom of God: but
unto them that are without, all these things are
done in parables" (v. 11). Then He continued,
"Know ye not this parable? and how then will ye
know all parables?" (v. 13).

Jesus was saying, "This is the key. If you gain
understanding of this parable, everything else
will start to open up to you."

Some people read the Bible and say, "I don't understand the Bible. It's Greek to me."

Well, the Bible was written in code form. That's why God gave us the Holy Ghost—to translate, interpret, and teach the Word to us. The reason many people have trouble understanding the Word is that they've never let the Holy Ghost be the teacher. They try to read the Bible with their own understanding.

But the Word is revelation truth. Verse 22 (AMP) says, "[Things are hidden temporarily only as a means to revelation.] For there is nothing hidden except to be revealed, nor is anything [temporarily] kept secret except in order that it may be made known." God's revelation truth was hidden not to keep it from us, but to keep it for us.

Every time you open your Bible, just ask the Holy Ghost to teach you. He is the Teacher of the Church, and He will reveal to you what is written on the pages.

———— ℘ ————

*Confession:*

*The Holy Ghost is my Teacher. He teaches me hidden truths and wonderful mysteries as I read and meditate on God's Word. I am planting the Word in my heart, and it is bearing rich fruit.*

## *What Are You Believing?*

*...for of the abundance of the heart his mouth speaketh.*

*Luke 6:45*

You can sometimes find out why a person is struggling in faith just by listening to him for a few minutes. For instance, people have come up to me after being prayed for in a healing line and have said, "Well, I still have such-and-such in my body. I don't know why I can't get rid of it."

I want to say to them, "You just told me why you haven't gotten rid of your condition!" You see, they're believing they can't get rid of it.

I've had other folks say, "I never get healed. When someone prays for me, I never receive anything." These people receive nothing because nothing is exactly what they're believing for!

When people come to receive prayer, they ought to be saying, "I've come to get rid of these symptoms."

"What do you have?"

"Well, I don't 'have' anything, but the devil is trying to put symptoms of sickness on me. I've come to get rid of them. You lay hands on me in the name of Jesus, and I'll receive my healing!"

Not only can we locate other people's faith by their words, but we can also discover what we really believe as we listen to our own words. When things aren't working right, we must listen to what we say.

Our words are important. If we can get our thinking, our believing, and our speaking straightened out, our lives will get straightened out. It may not happen instantly, but it will come to pass!

———— ✣ ————

*Confession:*

*I change my thinking, my believing,*
*and my speaking by feeding on God's Word.*
*As I think, believe, and speak God's truth,*
*His Word changes every area of my life!*

## *Enter Into Rest*

*For only we who believe God can enter into his place of rest.*

*Hebrews 4:3 (TLB)*

When you're in a difficult situation and you need a miracle, locate what you believe. Do you believe what God's Word says? Or do you believe what people or circumstances say?

Hebrews 4:3 says, "We which have believed do enter into rest." Belief produces rest, and what you hear determines what you believe.

So if you see you haven't entered into the rest of faith, don't waste your time feeling condemned, discouraged, or upset about it. Just realize your belief isn't yet strong enough to produce rest.

What do you do? Find out what the Word of God says about your situation. Search for

Scriptures that cover your case. Feed on the Word at every opportunity because hearing produces belief.

Some people say, "Well, when I have time, I'll do that." But if you maintain that attitude, you'll never have time.

If you need healing, listen to good healing tapes again and again. Read good books on healing, such as *Christ the Healer* by F. F. Bosworth. Don't just read the books once and set them down; read them from cover to cover several times until you are full of the Word on healing. Then out of the abundance of your heart, your mouth will speak. (Matt. 12:34.) You'll find yourself saying, "It's so good to be healed!"

And when someone asks, "Do you feel better? Are the symptoms gone?" you'll say "I haven't checked yet, but I know I'm healed because the Bible says it. I don't care what anybody says. God says healing is mine, and I have whatever God says!"

Remember, hearing produces belief, belief produces rest, and the rest of faith produces results!

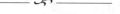

*Confession:*
*The Word of God is firmly lodged down*
*in my heart, and I enter into rest.*
*God's Word is greater inside me than*
*what I see with my natural eye.*
*It's so good to be healed!*

# PRAYER OF SALVATION

God loves you—no matter who you are, no matter what your past. God loves you so much that He gave His one and only begotten Son for you. The Bible tells us that "…whoever believes in him shall not perish but have eternal life" (John 3:16 NIV). Jesus laid down His life and rose again so that we could spend eternity with Him in heaven and experience His absolute best on earth. If you would like to receive Jesus into your life, say the following prayer out loud and mean it from your heart.

*Heavenly Father, I come to You admitting that I am a sinner. Right now, I choose to turn away from sin, and I ask You to cleanse me of all unrighteousness. I believe that Your Son, Jesus, died on the cross to take away my sins. I also believe that He rose again from the dead so that I might be forgiven of my sins and made righteous through faith in Him. I call upon the name of Jesus Christ to be the Savior and Lord of my life. Jesus, I choose to follow You and ask that You fill me with the power of the Holy Spirit. I declare that right now I am a child of God. I am free from sin and full of the righteousness of God. I am saved in Jesus' name. Amen.*

If you prayed this prayer to receive Jesus Christ as your Savior for the first time, please contact us on the web at **www.harrisonhouse.com** to receive a free book.

Or you may write to us at
**Harrison House**
P.O. Box 35035
Tulsa, Oklahoma 74153

## ABOUT THE AUTHOR

Mark Brazee has traveled to the nations since 1975 with a vision to reach the world with the truth of God's Word and the power of the Spirit. Mark and his wife, Janet, have traveled to more than 35 countries sharing the Good News of Jesus Christ and the overcoming life of faith.

Today, Mark Brazee Ministries spans the world through international DOMATA Ministers' Training Schools, as well as a stateside DOMATA School of Missions. Their broad scope of media outreaches include books, teaching tapes, music tapes, television, a quarterly magazine, and an internet Web site.

Mark and Janet Brazee also pastor World Outreach Church in Tulsa Oklahoma, where they base their outreach to the world.

To contact Mark Brazee,
please write to:

**Mark Brazee Ministries**
P.O. Box 1870
Broken Arrow, Oklahoma 74013-1870

Or visit us on the Web at:
www.brazee.org

*Please include your prayer requests
and comments when you write.*

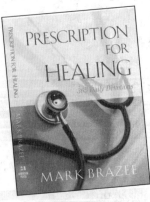

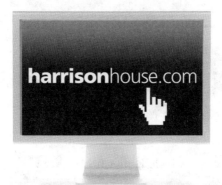

THE HARRISON HOUSE VISION

Proclaiming the truth and the power

Of the Gospel of Jesus Christ

With excellence;

Challenging Christians to

Live victoriously,

Grow spiritually,

Know God intimately.